Merry Christmas

with love & gratitude

to City Wellness staff

and teachers who provide

us with Peace, Joy, comfort

thru out the Years!

Many more blessings

to you all.

Marijane

Published by Willow Creek Press, Inc.
P.O. Box 147, Minocqua, Wisconsin 54548

Design: Donnie Rubo
Printed in China

COW
YOGA®

COW
YOGA®

WILLOW CREEK PRESS®

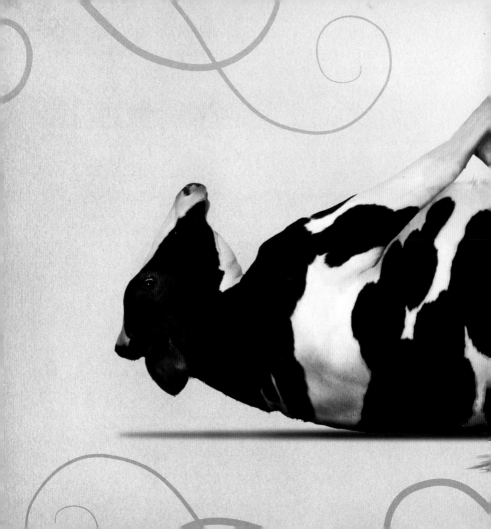

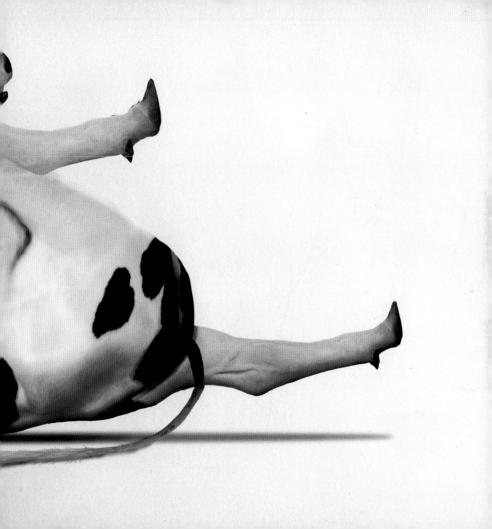

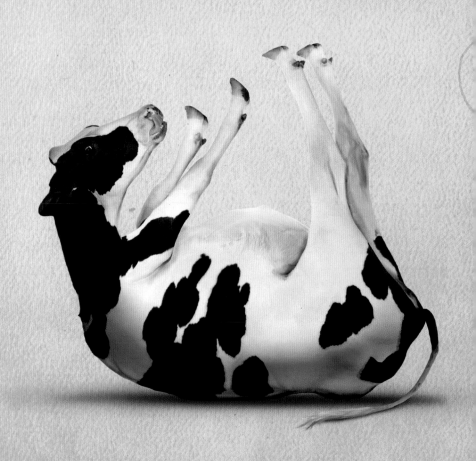

You only lose what you cling to.

—Buddha

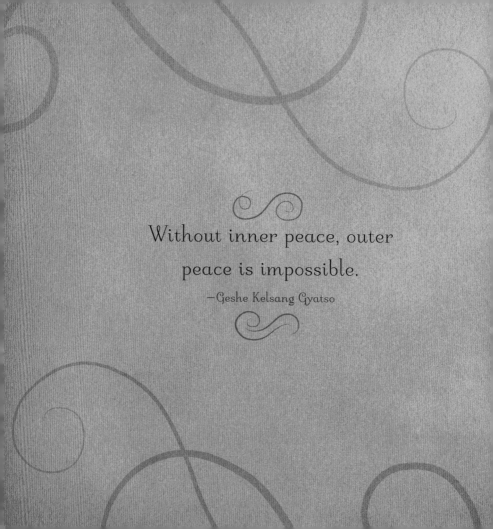

Without inner peace, outer peace is impossible.

—Geshe Kelsang Gyatso

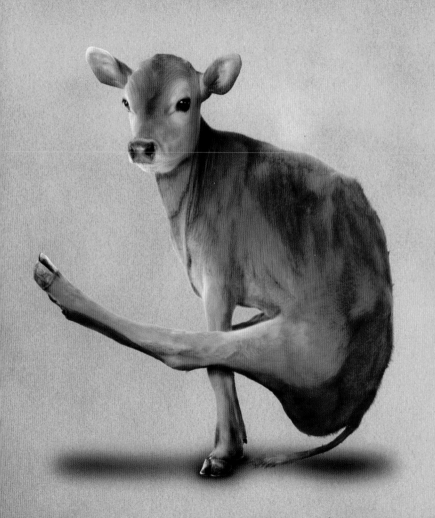

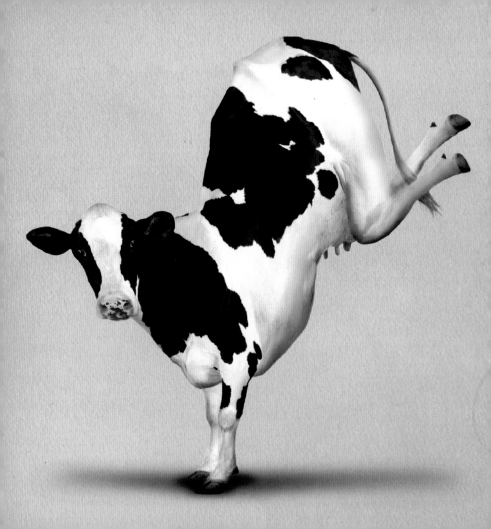

When you find peace within yourself,
you become the kind of person who
can live at peace with others.

—Peace Pilgrim

Your task is not to seek for love,
but merely to seek and find all
the barriers within yourself that
you have built against it.

—Rumi

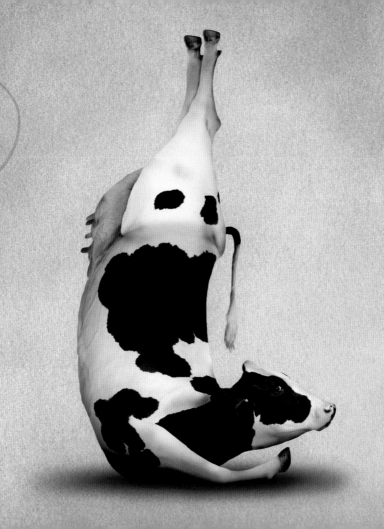

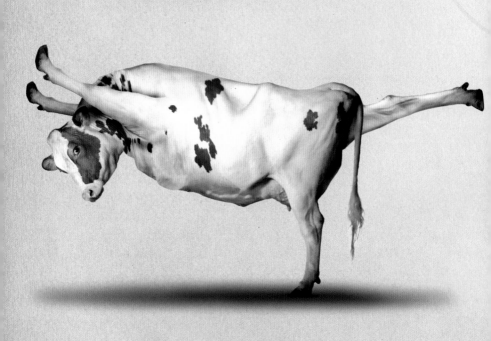

Silence is not silent. Silence speaks. It speaks most eloquently. Silence is not still. Silence leads. It leads most perfectly.

—Sri Chinmoy

Sun salutations can energize and warm you, even on the darkest, coldest winter day.

—Carol Krucoff

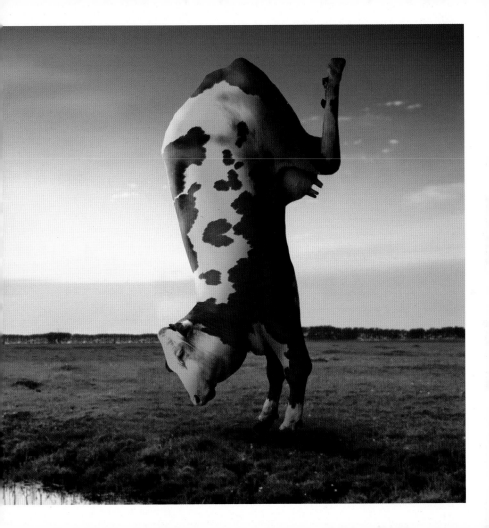

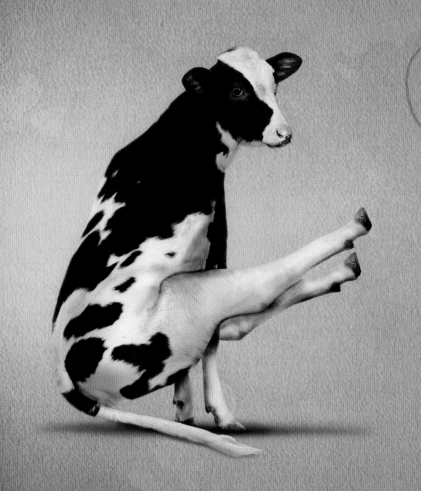

Mindfulness helps you go home to the present. And every time you go there and recognize a condition of happiness that you have, happiness comes.

—Thich Nhat Hanh

Better than a thousand hollow
words, is one word that brings peace.

—Buddha

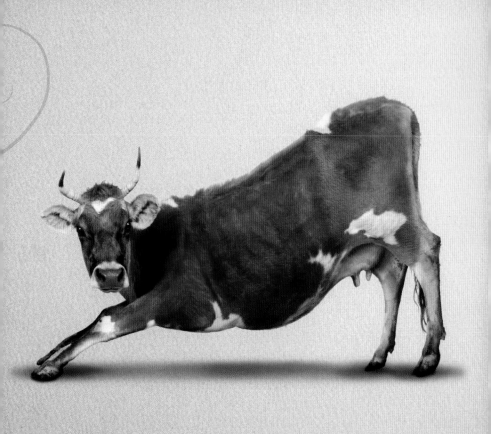

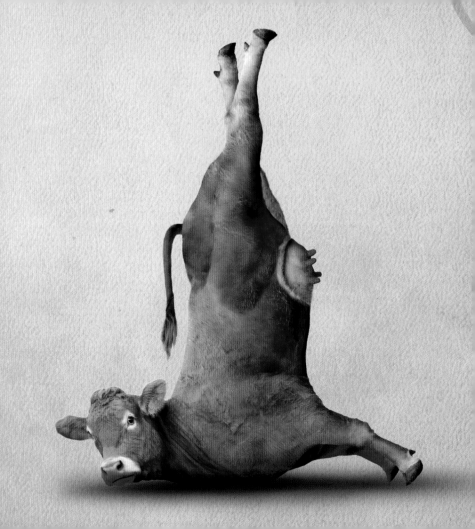

There is no need for temples, no
need for complicated philosophies.
My brain and my heart are my temples;
my philosophy is kindness.

—Dalai Lama

The part can never be well

unless the whole is well.

–Plato

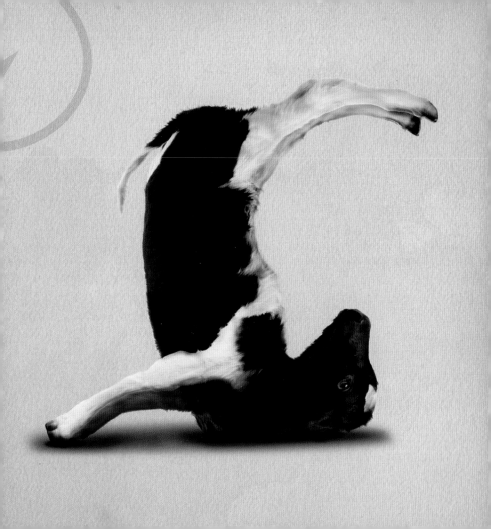

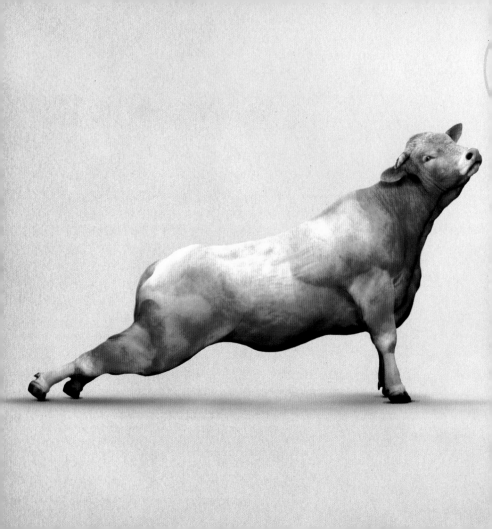

You must find the place inside yourself
where nothing is impossible.

—Deepak Chopra

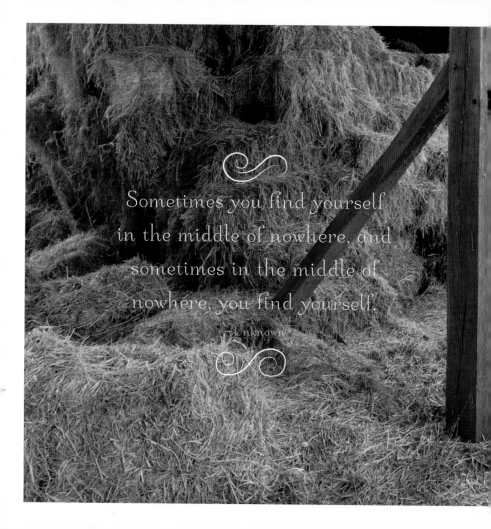

Sometimes you find yourself
in the middle of nowhere, and
sometimes in the middle of
nowhere, you find yourself.

—Unknown

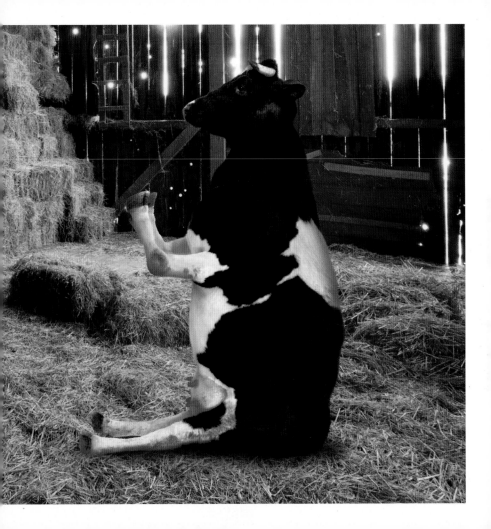

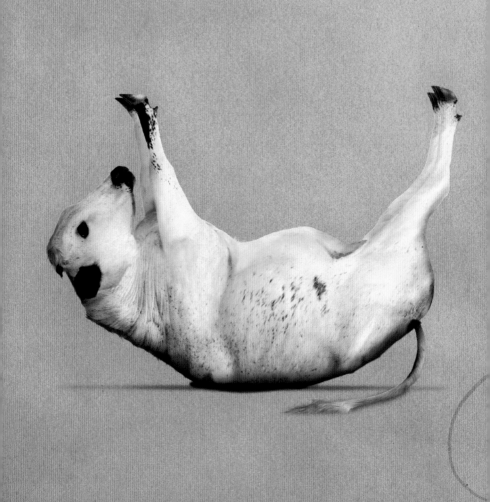

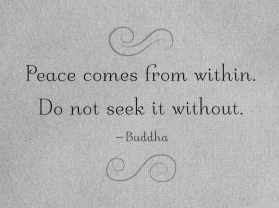

Peace comes from within.
Do not seek it without.

—Buddha

Our bodies are our gardens to
which our wills are gardeners.

—William Shakespeare

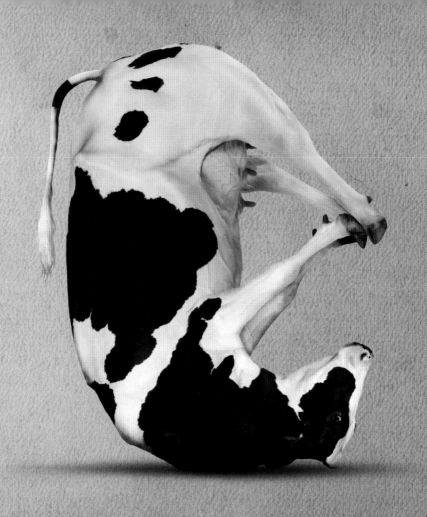

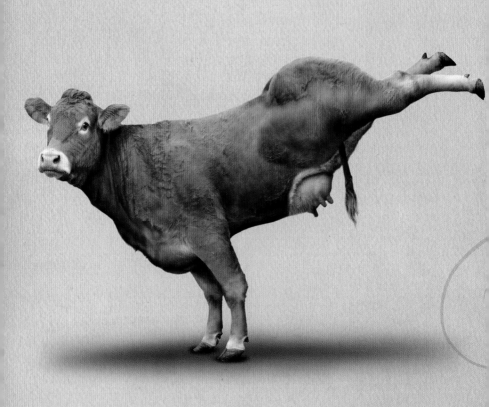

A river cuts through a rock, not because
of its power, but its persistence.

–Unknown

Blessed are the flexible, for they
shall not be bent out of shape.

—Unknown

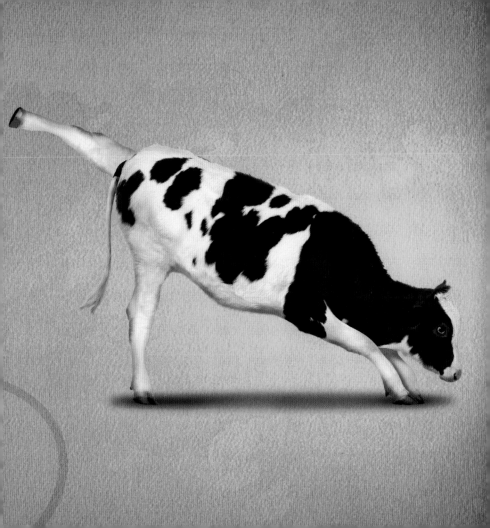

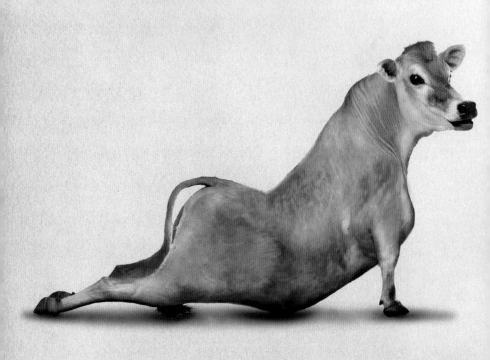

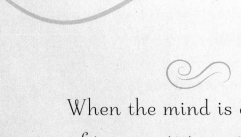

When the mind is exhausted
of images, it invents its own.

—Gary Snyder

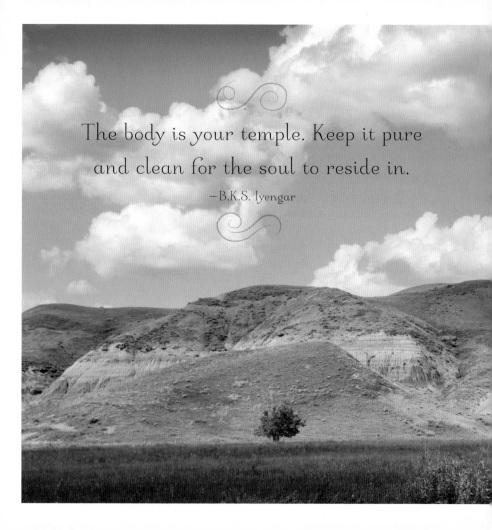

The body is your temple. Keep it pure
and clean for the soul to reside in.

–B.K.S. Iyengar

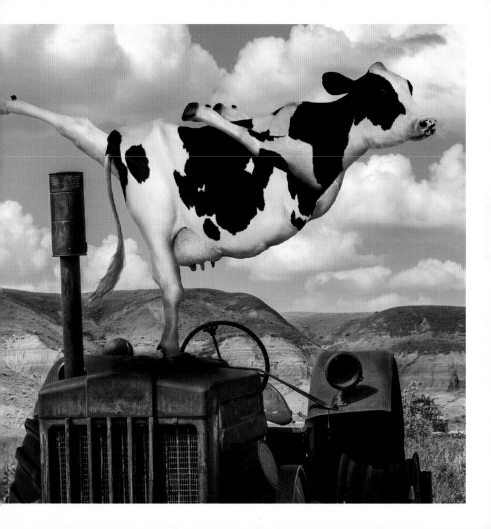

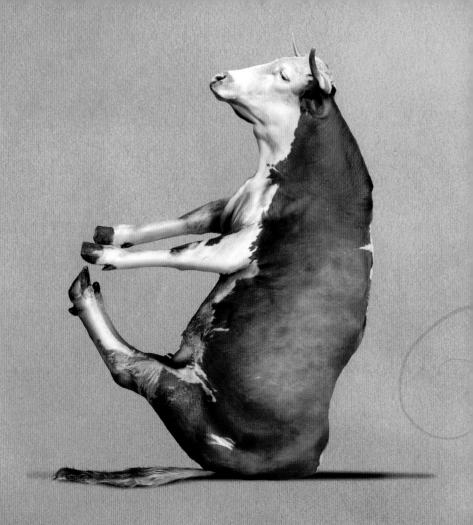

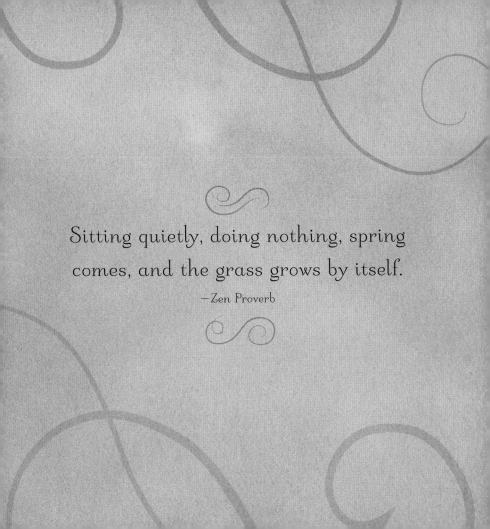

Sitting quietly, doing nothing, spring comes, and the grass grows by itself.

—Zen Proverb

The wise man lets go of all results,
whether good or bad, and is
focused on the action alone.

—Bhagavad Gita

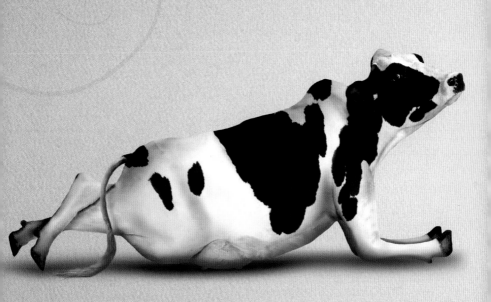

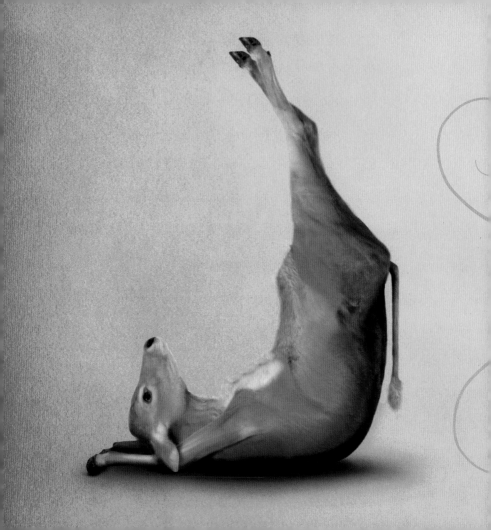

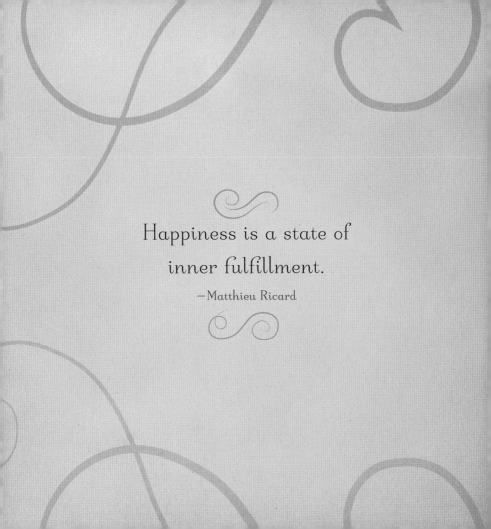

Happiness is a state of
inner fulfillment.

—Matthieu Ricard

Yoga is like music. The rhythm of
the body, the melody of the mind,
and the harmony of the soul
create the symphony of life.

—B.K.S. Iyengar

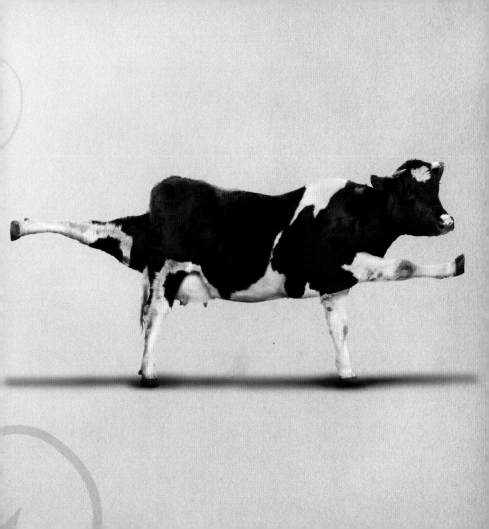

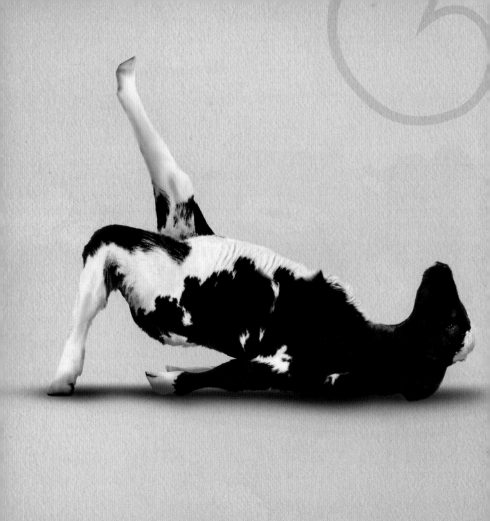

Have wisdom in your actions

and faith in your merits.

—Yogi Bhajan

Happiness is not a matter of intensity but of balance, order, rhythm and harmony.

—Thomas Merton

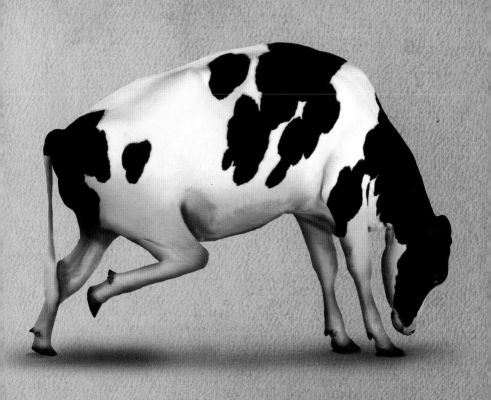

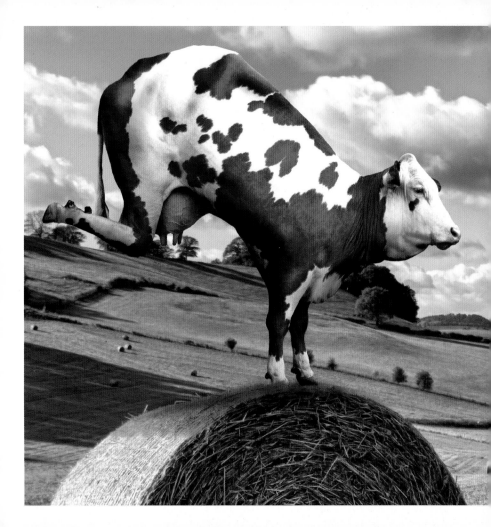

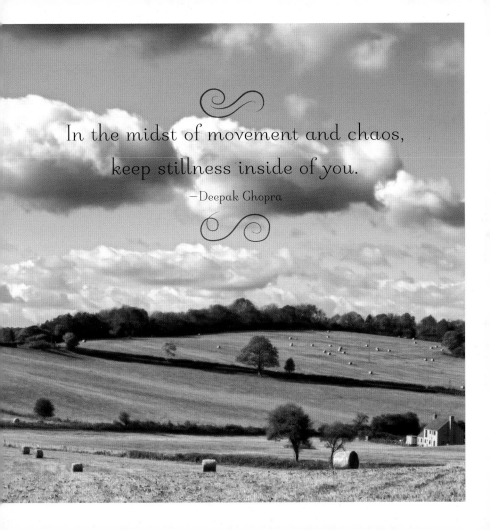

In the midst of movement and chaos,
keep stillness inside of you.

—Deepak Chopra

In our uniquely human capacity of
connect movement with breath and
spiritual meaning, yoga is born.

—Gurmukh Kaur Khalsa

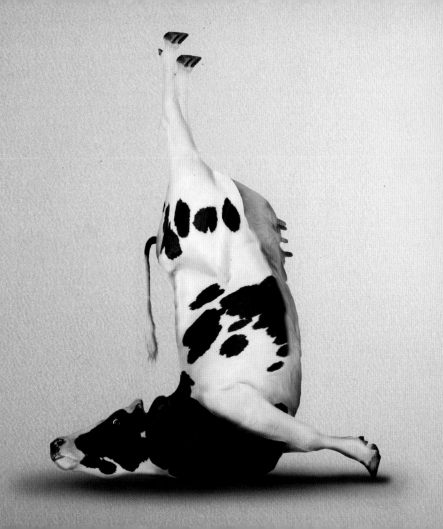

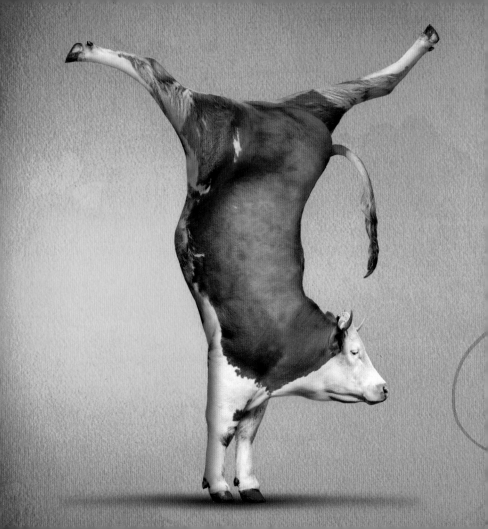

Out of your vulnerabilities

will come your strength.

—Sigmund Freud

The quieter you become the
more you are able to hear.

−Rumi

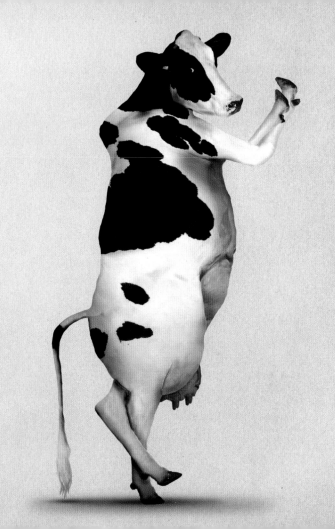

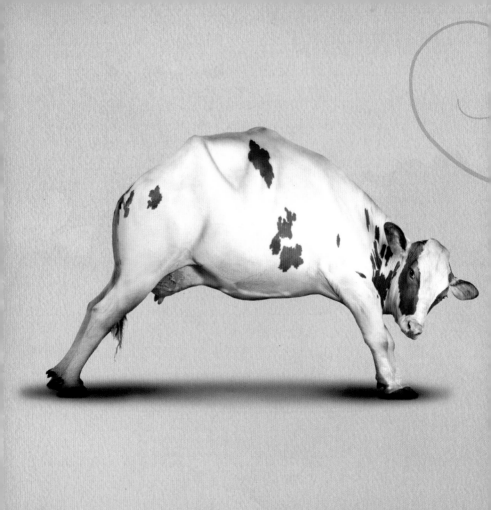

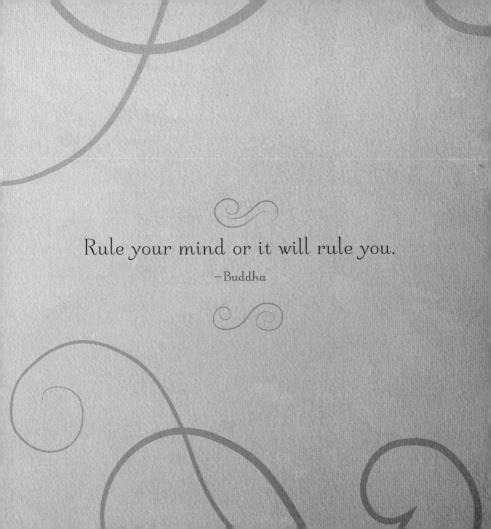

Rule your mind or it will rule you.

—Buddha

Do not feel lonely, the entire universe is inside you.

–Rumi

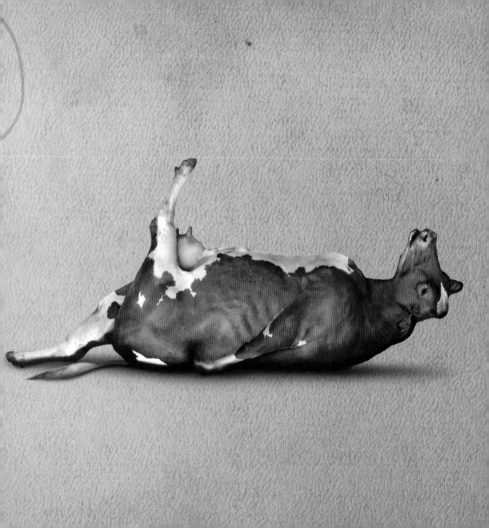

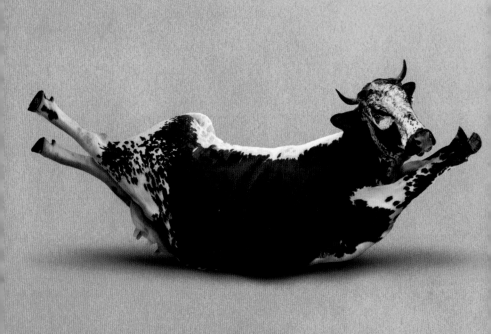

What lies behind us and what lies
before us are tiny matters compared
to what lies within us.

—Ralph Waldo Emerson

What we think, we become.

—Buddha

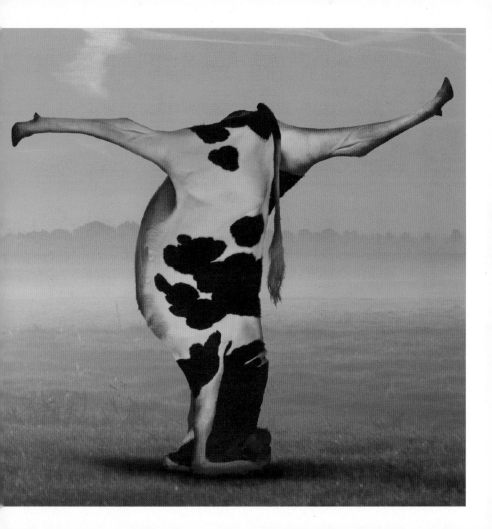

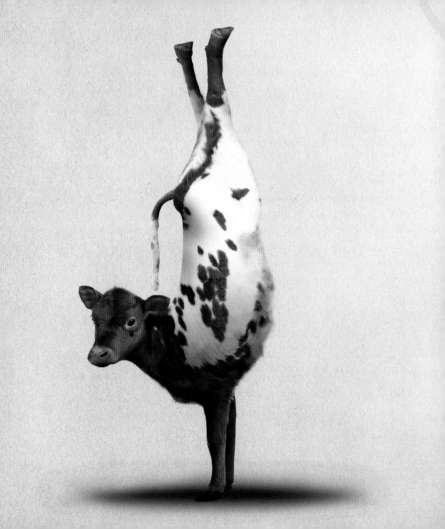

True happiness is to learn how
to live beyond the imperfections.

—Rita Maatta

The End